AF413715

FOOLING MY FERTILITY & EXPECTING AT 50

How I Had A Baby in Midlife & You Can Too

Disclaimer: I am not a doctor, everything in this book is what contributed to
my success while working in close consultation with my team of doctors. Before
taking any of the supplements or actions I undertook, consult your doctors for
their professional recommendations.

To my precious baby boy MMG, so happy you are here; life is better with you! To my family and friends who are still supporting me, I could not have done it without you!

And to you, Dear Reader, by reading this book, you are actively opening the door for new possibilities in your life. I wish you the Very Best.

CONTENTS

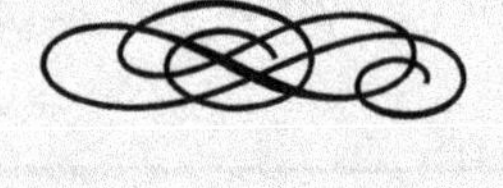

SECTION

One

PRE-PREGNANCY

On Mindset

Once we accept the idea that everyone has their own unique journey to motherhood, we can release the woulda, coulda, shouldas that hinder us. Yes, you may be older now than you were, but I believe that if God could do it for Sarah and Abraham in the Bible (Genesis 17:15-19), then He can do it for you, too. God is no respecter of persons. If He can do it for me, He can do it for you. Whether you get pregnant naturally, with IVF, with donor assistance, surrogate assistance, or adopt, accept the basic idea that Motherhood is definitely happening. With that decision made and accepted, watch how many avenues will open up to you, and how quickly your circumstances will begin to change.

How I Got Here and Why I Waited This Long

Like many young girls, I grew up playing "Mommy and Baby" with my dolls. I also loved to read books and sing along with my Barbie transistor radio. I always knew that I wanted to be a mother from age 5, and I never thought it would be difficult to achieve. In my mind it was a given. I never had any doubt about it. It was only in my adult years when my body was not cooperating, that I was faced with the incredible realization that it was easier for me to get cast in musicals and TV shows than it was for me to get pregnant. How crazy was that?

I come from a foundational American family. My mother's side of the family comes from Virginia and North Carolina, and my father's side of the family comes from the South Carolina Lowcountry. On both sides, they worked the land growing cash crops as slaves and later as sharecroppers. My family worked hard over the centuries so that each succeeding generation could have more, do better and run faster. There was a particular story that my grandmother used to tell us about her time working in a seaside motel as a chambermaid. A guest went out of his way to come give her a tip and it was a penny cut in half. Can you imagine working long, hot, back-breaking hours to have someone come place a half of a penny into your hand with a smirk? Nevertheless, she persevered. Both of my grandmothers did everything for me. Honestly, there was nothing I wanted or needed growing up that they didn't provide. Impressive, for women who only completed the 3rd and 6th grades respectively.

So it was no surprise that when I was born, the edict from the women in my family that I heard early and often was, "don't bring no babies home!". I knew that if I got pregnant as a teenager or as an unmarried person my mother was going take me out of here, and I had big plans for my life. I took it very seriously when they said not to bring any babies home! I remained a virgin until I was 18 years old. College was busy, with more studies than sex, but the year after I graduated college and moved back home to Atlanta, I did get caught out, and I found myself pregnant from a casual relationship. I was broke as broke could be, living in the basement of a house in Midtown with two other girls while waiting tables for two dollars and forty cents per hour plus tips. I didn't see any way to make that work. Reluctantly, I terminated my pregnancy, which was in my current estimation, one of the biggest mistakes I ever made. I often look back and wonder how my life would've been different had I carried that child to term. I often wonder, too, if in my adulthood, I subconsciously thought perhaps that I didn't deserve any children because I terminated that pregnancy. It's possible, that I held that belief deep in my subconscious thoughts, but that is a mental paradigm that I have thankfully done away with.

Career Over Everything

There was an expectation in the family that I would become a doctor. After all, I majored in chemistry at the number six institution in the nation. So of course I went on to further disappoint the family by interning at Rowdy Records under the helm of Dallas Austin and Clive Davis. I joined a girl group for a few years, then jumped into musical theater traveling all across the country doing shows, and then moved to LA to chase my television dreams. By the time I transitioned into the business of entertainment, and started working corporately, two decades had passed by. I was still chasing a decent paycheck. I was still trying to figure out my personal life. My family had thrown up their hands. They didn't understand any of the choices I had made, and if I am being honest, they were pretty disappointed in how things had panned out for me and by extension, for them. But hey, at least I didn't bring no babies home, so there's that.

Failing at Egg Freezing

By age 40, I had been on and off of birth control for about 20 years. In my 20s I only had one serious relationship and that did not end in marriage, so no babies were brought home. When I turned 39 I had my second serious relationship which evolved into an engagement quickly within three months. I thought that I might still be young enough to try to get pregnant, but that engagement ended and so thus again, no babies were brought home. Shortly after that, I had another relationship and as we were heading towards engagement, I had a girlfriend who had frozen her eggs at 40 years old. She told me about the process which sounded super easy. I knew that this relationship was going to be slower moving because my partner was in the entertainment industry like me and didn't want to slow down his life for children. Our compromise was for me to freeze my eggs.

I got off of the pill about 3 months before I was ready to freeze so that my ovaries could get used to working normally again. I borrowed money at a highway robbery interest rate and happily went to see my friend's IVF doctor in Encino, California to start my egg freezing process. I thought it would be straightforward and easy because it flowed easily for my friend; however, that was not the case for me. After an initial examination, the doctor told me I had fibroids, which I already knew but that should not be an impediment to egg freezing and could be dealt with later. I started the injections to grow my follicles for the egg freezing procedure and as I began traveling back and forth to the office, visit after visit, nothing was happening. There were 0 follicles in one ovary and 1 follicle in the other. The doctor asked me what I wanted to do. Did I want to harvest what we could from the one follicle and come back every month to harvest one or more follicles? I was confused. I wasn't sure if he was asking me did I want to spend $8k every month to harvest one follicle, because he said it like it was the most logical thing in the world. So I asked him to clarify and he said yes, he was indeed asking me if this is what I wanted to do. Ha! I told him no. Emphatically. I decided to cut short the egg freezing process since I had not finished paying for it and it was clear that I was probably not going to get a good egg from the one follicle. I went home, drank a bottle of red wine and cried myself to sleep.

It was after that that my doctor decided to test my FSH (follicle-stimulating hormone) and AMH (anti-müllerian hormone) which we probably should have done at the beginning. I was diagnosed with Diminished Ovarian Reserve and I began entertaining the idea in my mind that I had run out of eggs. This was very hard to fathom as I have always been exceptionally healthy, youthful and focused on eating well. I didn't understand how all the other parts of my body were in perfect working order except for my reproductive system.

I arrived at the theory that taking the birth control pill for decades had suppressed my ovaries and they were never going to bounce back. This was in fact, untrue. As I got off of the pill and stayed off, a year or two later, when I went in to my gynecologist for ultrasounds, we could visualize multiple follicles on both sides. With that I began to think, well, I'll just meet someone and get pregnant naturally.

Fibroids

"Meeting someone" proved a lot more difficult than I thought, and when I did, the men either didn't want kids, had had a vasectomy, already had kids, were not as single as they presented themselves to be, and the whole thing was just a nightmare. I also still had the issue of the fibroids looming over my head. My IVF doctor would not let me do IUI or insemination due to the fibroids. He wanted me to have a myomectomy first. I didn't want to have surgery for a couple of reasons. I knew too many women who had had multiple fibroid surgeries, because each time they had the surgery, the fibroids would be back within a year.

Most doctors will tell you that they don't quite know what causes fibroids. What we do know is that they grow by having an influx of too much estrogen, but fibroids are definitely more prevalent in black women than they are in women of other races and nationalities. According to the University of Michigan Health Lab, "Nearly a quarter of Black women between 18 and 30 have fibroids compared to about 6% of white women, according to some national estimates. By age 35, that number increases to 60%. Black women are also two to three times more likely to have recurring fibroids or suffer from complications."[1] Many black women have anecdotally come to the conclusion that it comes from carrying a lot of

---

1   https://www.michiganmedicine.org/health-lab/understanding-racial-disparities-women-uterine-fibroids

survival related stress, pressure, and emotion with no outlet for that energy.

Regardless, I was still in the heat of the battle in trying to create a career and a life for myself. I was trying to earn at a level that would even make me able to sustain having a family, and I had the feeling that if I had a surgery the fibroids would return right away because I didn't know how to change my lifestyle in terms of stress management. Also, I didn't think I would be able to take two months off of work, which is what you would need for recovering from the myomectomy if you have the C-section incision, and I didn't have that much vacation time or sick time. I didn't want to be fired from my underpaying job, so that was always an obstacle for me. I didn't see a way for me to move forward with surgery and I was nervous about it so I started looking into natural ways to get rid of my fibroids such as acupuncture, Chinese herbs, prayer and meditation. My fibroids were already too big for these to be effective, but I didn't realize that until about 8 years later.

Then to add insult to injury, as time went on I also would have cysts pop up on my ovaries from time to time and my periods became more and more heavy. We are talking wearing two and three nighttime maxi pads at a time, heavy. I was passing huge blood clots half the size of my palm. I initially thought that the heavy bleeding and the clots were a function of the fibroids, but they were also a function of my hormones being out of whack because I was in perimenopause and did not know it. I should have been able to put it together since I had already been diagnosed with diminished ovarian reserve, but I try to be an optimist. And honestly, I was still thinking that I would possibly just pop up pregnant naturally at some point because I have faith in God's promises. As it turns out, I did eventually pop up pregnant, but I could not have even begun to imagine exactly how that would happen.

Adoption

I moved from Los Angeles back to the New York metro area in 2018 and had taken a sales job that was even more stressful than the jobs I had previously. The trade off however, was that they paid substantially more than I had ever earned, so I was holding on for dear life. Now, I was definitely making enough money to parent a child on my own and support a great lifestyle, but with Covid I wasn't dating, and with my job there wasn't really time anyway. I was working at a startup and we were scrambling to survive during the early days of Covid, so I was working up to 18 hour days. I had essentially accepted the fact that pregnancy was not going to happen for me.

At this point I was looking toward fostering or adopting through the state. So I began my research, doing my Google-ations and found that the state of New Jersey, where I happened to live was not accepting any new applicants for fostering or adopting. It was a very curious situation because I know there were a lot of children locked at home 24 hours a day with their stressed-out parents, and some of these children were probably being abused. Normally these kids would be identified by a teacher at school and moved into a foster situation, so I was wondering what was happening to these kids? It seems as though the state was more worried about putting the kids into a home where there was Covid and the kids possibly dying from Covid, than the abuse the kids might be suffering at home. This was the very early days of Covid, so for a time, it was understandable, but this went on for nearly 2 ½, almost 3 years. I waited a few months to see if they would open up the process because certainly doing it through the state was going to be more cost-effective than going through private adoption, but waiting for the state to open back up was taking too long, so I started looking for private adoption agencies.

I found one in Philadelphia that works with expecting mothers throughout the tri-state area so I thought I had a good chance of matching with an expectant mother of my background. Going through all of the classes and creating my adoption book, which is a picture book of my life and my "village" that the child would be adopted into took about a year. Then finally, I was on the list of waiting families which was a very exciting day I have to say. Rather quickly I was selected by a young expecting mother. She was 16 and she had an interesting reason for choosing me. She did not want the child to experience any more loss so she thought that if a single woman adopted the child and later married a man, "when the man leaves" that the child would always go with the adopting mother and not be a pawn in divorce, which was interesting and also a stinging commentary on the state of affairs in our society. I met the young lady and her young mother at a diner in central New Jersey. She was very lovely but I could tell that she was conflicted about going through with adoption. She had a lot of pressure from her mother to go through with it because at 16, she was far too young to be mothering. On the other hand, her father's side of the family wanted her to keep the child and they just couldn't imagine how she would even consider adoption as an option. Interestingly, her father's side of the family was not contributing anything to her life. It was her very young mother who was taking care of her and all of her siblings and who also ultimately would be the person to take care of this coming baby. Besides that shade of reluctance, we had a great meeting and then I went and bought all the stuff I would need for the baby on Amazon. Stroller, bassinet, bottles, linens, clothes, formula, everything the agency recommended I should have on deck as the young lady was due to deliver within a month. I met with my leadership at work to get a maternity leave of sorts worked out. I got the items home, got set up and waited as the young lady indicated that she wanted me to be at the hospital when she delivered. After some weeks I received a call from her caseworker saying that she had changed her mind. The pressure from her father's side of family had become too great and she decided to parent, which was completely understandable.

I waited the rest of that year for another phone call from my agency but no phone call was forthcoming. I met with my agency and they said that I was a little too picky on my family matching form about what I was willing to accept as it relates to how much drug and alcohol the expectant mother would have exposed herself to. I explained to them that as a single person I want to be able to provide the best for the child and a child who had a great deal of special needs would be difficult for me as an only parent. They said I needed to put yes next to every drug question on the form in order to get shown to more mothers. I had written WTC (willing to consider) next to each drug and that was putting me behind other families in the presentations. So needless to say I was growing a bit frustrated.

Myomectomy

At this time we were well into year two of Covid and in the startup I was working for. We were working super long days and making a ton of cash, but it was a very stressful business and as my stress levels grew, so did my fibroids to the point that it was just unbearable. It was hard to sit for long periods of time, and you could feel the fibroids when you touched my stomach. That's how big they were. So after many years of trying to get rid of them with herbs and acupuncture I decided to finally start looking for a doctor to help me. I didn't want just anyone to perform my myomectomy. I knew from all of the experiences that I had heard my friends go through over the last 10 years that I would need a very specific doctor who had wide experience with large fibroids as well as endometriosis because I thought that might be an issue for me as well.

What I did was, I actually googled for an endometriosis doctor and I found one who had a large number of Google reviews. The women were raving about the surgery that he performed on them, and how he had removed all of the endo, and all of the fibroids. He sounded very promising. I called his office to make an appointment for a consultation late on a Friday afternoon. Saturday morning around 8 AM, I received a phone call from the doctor personally and we talked for a few minutes about my situation. He said that he thought he could help me and told me to make an appointment with his nurse. I went to see him the next week for the ultrasound and he was very confident that he could get rid of my fibroids. I asked him about his experience with black women and large intramuscular fibroids as that was my situation, and he told me about his more complicated cases. I had obgyns and fertility doctors want to perform the myomectomy on me previously, and that never sat right with me. I actually had one fertility doctor in North Jersey tell me in 2018 that my fibroids were too large and that she would give me a hysterectomy. I say all this to say that every doctor of women's medicine is not qualified to perform a myomectomy even though they may be certified to do so. The doctor that wanted to give me the hysterectomy didn't know how to perform the surgery so her default move was to take my reproductive organs altogether! Don't be afraid to challenge doctors in your consultations. If they get defensive, then that is not the doctor for you. This endometriosis/fibroid doctor that I had found *only* did this kind of surgery all day every day. He had seen every kind of disfigured uterus there is. He was ready to move quickly with me. If I'm being honest, that made me slightly nervous. He wanted to schedule the surgery for the next month which was December of 2021 but that was the middle of my busy season at work so we ended up scheduling it for January 2022. He kept saying that after he did the surgery on me that I would be able to carry a baby with no problem. I laughed at him because my period was highly irregular. At this point I was deep into perimeno-pause. I had no dating prospects and barely any eggs, so I didn't really see how it was going to happen for me, but nevertheless we moved forward. My surgeon uses the da Vinci surgical system. He goes in with the robot hands and excises the fibroids, cuts them into smaller pieces while still inside of the abdomen, then pulls them out through your belly button in a bag. It sounds wild, I know.

The surgery was a success, and I went home the same day. Recovery was not bad. Getting to the point where I could walk around my home and do the bare minimum like heating up food in a microwave and going to the restroom, only took about a week, but I was so depleted from my job that I took three weeks to rest. My uterus was finally back to normal. I had space in my abdomen again. I didn't always have pressure on my bladder anymore. I could sleep through the night without pee breaks and I felt much lighter. My doctor said that I should wait 6 to 8 months and then if I wanted to get pregnant, I could. Again, I was laughing at him because I just had no idea how that would ever happen, even with a nearly perfect womb.

Embryo Adoption

I refocused on travel and work that year to take my mind off of the fact that I had not had any other offers for adoption. At the end of the year, I began looking around at other adoption agencies and reading their newsletters as I was becoming more frustrated. In one of the newsletters I saw mention of embryo adoption. Embryo adoption is the opportunity to "adopt" and implant unused embryos from a couple or a woman who knows that they will not be able to use all of the ones they have created in their IVF journey, but they do not want them destroyed or donated to science. The owners of these embryos will donate them to various agencies for other families who cannot get pregnant, to adopt these embryos and use them in their own IVF cycle. Or, they will go into an embryo program at the clinic where they were created to be used with other patients at that clinic. Or, sometimes embryo donation is person-to-person, where the donor family meets the recipient family on a message board or Facebook group or knows them in real life, and they organize the donation together through their respective clinics. This was all new to me! Obviously, I knew that I could obtain donor eggs and donor sperm and make embryos on my own, but this would be costly. It can cost up to $30k to get an egg donor. Sperm donations are not that expensive, but you still have to pay to create the embryos which can be in the neighborhood of $10,00 to $15,000. When you adopt an embryo, all of that is already done and the cost to create the embryos is often not reflected in the cost for you to adopt them. I'd never heard of adopting an embryo that had already been created, but it seemed like an absolutely perfect solution to my problems. I know that parents who create several embryos sometimes come to realize that they can't afford to parent all of those children, but don't want to destroy the embryos and don't want to donate them to science and are just generally con-flicted about what to do with them. And then there are people like me who have hesitancy about creating embryos and there being a possibility that none of those embryos would be viable. That would have been too devastating to me after all of my failed egg freezing from a decade before. I liked the fact that through the IVF clinic that created these embryos, they had already been tested for genetic diseases and had a high quality grade, so I began mulling this over in my mind. Could this really be an option for me? I reached back out to my fibroid surgeon to ask him if I could indeed do IVF, and he said yes, so at that point I started investigating all of the steps in the process to adopt an embryo.

I reached out to the traditional adoption agency which also operates the embryo adoption agency and published this newsletter, and they were very responsive and polite, but when they found out that I was single and 49 they said that they could not work with me. They gave me some other referrals and I ended up inquiring with several agencies. A second agency was also very polite, but they said they don't get very many African-American embryos, so finally I had narrowed down the situation to a clinic in California where I would actually have to go there in person to do the whole process, which I was open to since I was working remotely. But then I found another agency in Tennessee that had diverse background embryos, no rules against my age or marital status and would ship to my local IVF clinic. I identified the embryos I wanted. I was able to see a picture of each anonymous donor and the testing they had been through, the medical background of their family members, and in some cases they even answered some questions about why they chose to be donors which I thought would all be very helpful to share with my children as a part of their origin story. I read to my son the book of his origin story a few times a week, similar to what I had planned to do with any child I had adopted traditionally. I have four brothers myself and one of them is adopted. He always knew he was adopted, it was never a secret, nor was it a big deal. It was just a fact like many other facts about our family. Unfortunately, the agency I adopted from sadly is no longer in business but is by no means the only option for women 50 and over. You will find a list of resources at the end of this book.

Choosing An IVF Doctor

With my embryos chosen and secured, I started looking for an IVF doctor. I think it's important to not select an IVF clinic based on perhaps the good experiences a friend of yours had, or the things you've heard, but it's important to pick the right doctor within a particular clinic for *you* because you've already checked their reviews about their bedside manner, and you can identify people who have had a successful process with them. I did three consultations at three different IVF clinics before I made my final decision, and I'm glad that I did because at the end of all of that, I was very clear on what the game plan was going to be. I was clear on timelines. I believed the doctor I selected had the best game plan, and that he wasn't just rushing me into a frozen embryo transfer (FET) as a money grab, without first prepping the uterus for the best possible outcome.

I went through the same process of selection that I did when I chose my myomectomy surgeon. I had a list of questions I wanted to ask to ensure we were on the same page and that the odds would be leaning toward a positive outcome. After having different embryo agencies tell me that they couldn't work with me because I was not married or because I was 49 years old, that became the primary question that I had of these various clinics. Do they work with single women? Do they work with women who are my age? Is there a cut off age that they won't work with? What would the possible complications be? Some places are very rigid about it and other places are not.

I know that people have a lot of opinions about this, but what is important to me is that my child has a good life and a large village. Young parents unfortunately pass away every day, even more so now than before the COVID-19 pandemic. And if I had been an unhealthy person, and had not had grandparents who lived into their 90s and parents who are still alive today at almost 80, then perhaps I would not have done it. But with humility, I knew that my 50 is like someone else's 35. I made a practical and financial plan for my children should anything ever happen to me. And then I turned my attention toward giving a child a great life. Usually when you have IVF doctors that are in a city center or a metropolis, they are used to women who have waited to have children because of their careers into their 40s and 50s or who have been trying unsuccessfully for years. It's not unusual for them to have women coming to them in their 50s trying to get pregnant. But that isn't true of *every* clinic, even in the New York City metro area.

One clinic was really interesting. They will work with people from anywhere around the globe through their "care from anywhere" program. You do all of your initial ultrasounds at home with their remote access equipment and bloodwork at Labcorp through their exclusive partnership, or with a local clinic if needed, and then when it is time to do the actual frozen embryo transfer, you either do it at your local partner clinic or fly to New York to their flagship clinic. I found this clinic because of the doctor who founded it. He had amazing reviews all over Google from two different clinics he had previously worked for in the NYC metro area, and I wanted to work with him specifically. However, due to the fact that this clinic offers bespoke service, the pricing was a bit more than I wanted to pay. I also looked at other clinics that were big franchise type clinics with lower pricing, but I did an incredible amount of research on the specific doctors at these clinics. This was hours of research, looking up reviews on each doctor's name at these clinics and working to pinpoint a doctor that I thought would be well disposed towards me. In this case, the larger franchise clinic was just not for me. The google reviews weren't bad, but it seemed as though there were just so many women in and out of their offices for bloodwork and appointments that it might affect my availability for work in the mornings. Also from what I read, it didn't seem like there was a personalized feel to their service. I then I found a clinic that was smaller, with a philosophy of giving women "more." They seemed as though they cared about women and had a lovely pink office. When I went there however, the woman who was doing my initial blood work and intake questions was looking at me like I had two heads because I was single, 49 and trying to get pregnant. She literally looked incredulous as she asked me about my plans. I did not feel comfortable there. I ended up selecting one of the clinics that the fabulously reviewed doctor was working with at the time he opened his "care from anywhere" clinic. It was not the biggest, and was certainly not the most fancy in terms of waiting rooms and amenities. It was actually very basic looking, just like a basic doctors office. However, they treated me like any other normal woman who is going through the process, and they had a smart and specific plan of action for me. At the time I was undertaking this, I had not had a period in about 12 months which my nurse practitioner told me was "officially" menopause. So my doctor's plan was to wake up my uterus by doing a month of hormones to trigger a period shed. They also ran my blood work numerous times to make sure that everything was looking good in terms of my blood counts, hemoglobin, and iron to see how well I would be able to support this pregnancy. This plan made sense to me, and I felt confident in it, so ultimately, I selected them.

I wanted to be sure to ask them all of the questions that I had at each consultation, so aside from my "do you work with women who are single", I also asked, do you see any fibroids that have come back? How does the uterus look in terms of embryo implantation? I asked a *litany* of questions around my blood work in the months leading up to the frozen embryo transfer. I have historically been anemic, so my RBC (red blood cells) and my WBC (white blood cells) were always of a high concern to me. Almost every reading in the CBC (complete blood count) blood work I asked questions about, especially if it wasn't in the normal range, according to Labcorp. If I wasn't in the normal range for a particular reading then I would Google that reading and then look for herbs or supplements I could take to get myself into the normal range. For instance, my first RBC reading was slightly under the range and I immediately purchased some liquid iron for faster absorption instead of taking iron tablets as I've always done my whole life. I was also looking at doing iron transfusions because I knew that I wanted to move quickly, but I asked the IVF doctor about that and he said no, I did not need to do transfusions as my iron was not that low. He said that the liquid iron should be sufficient. My white blood cell count was a little low as well and the IVF doctor didn't seem very concerned about it, but I was determined to leave no stone unturned before stepping into this frozen embryo transfer. I googled again, and found that the herb Cat's Claw is used by many people to support their immune systems and get the WBC back into normal range, so I purchased some on Amazon.

There is a website called Fertility IQ, https://www.fertilityiq.com/ that I used to research specific IVF doctors, and it was extremely enlightening as I was making a decision about which clinic to use. It was incredibly helpful in terms of real people sharing their honest experiences with these doctors, and it really helped me in terms of eliminating any indecision.

Choosing an OBGYN and an MFM

My IVF doctor said I had to have a clearance from my OB to make sure that I was in good health and able to carry a pregnancy to completion, so that's how this OB search began. The only doctor I had seen from the time I moved back to the East Coast from LA was my general practitioner, and I never even met her in person. The nurse practitioner was the only person working every time I visited that office. I had also seen that one previously mentioned fertility doctor right before the pandemic who immediately wanted to give me a hysterectomy and never even offered a myomectomy as a solution. Glad I didn't listen to her! Doctors like her are the precise reason it is so important to vet, research and interview your prospective doctors. They don't all have the same wealth of knowledge and experience. When it comes to fibroids, the ones who are not experienced often just want to take your womb and keep things moving. If that is not what you want, then I implore you to say no and find someone else.

As I was newly relocated back to the East Coast, I had to start from zero finding an OB/GYN who would be suitable to team up with my IVF doctor. The first OB I went to was very inspirational because she was 54, had her first child as a single mother at age 50, and had her second child at age 52. I felt so fortunate to meet her, almost like God was sending me a little message to keep going, through her. She was very supportive of what I was trying to do. However, this particular OB worked in several different offices and due to how awesome she was, she was always swamped. It always took an hour past my appointment time to get in to see her. With the nature of her overcrowded appointment schedule, and multiple offices, I knew that there was a high likelihood of her not being available to deliver my baby so I decided not to stay with her despite how inspirational I found her to be.

The second OB I had was a man, and he was great. There were no weird vibes, nor did he make me feel bad in any way about what I was undertaking. He was very clear and upfront about the fact that he thought I needed to have a C-section because my pregnancy was high risk, due to the fact that it was an IVF baby and two, because I already had incisions in my uterus during the myomectomy which would put me and the baby at risk for uterine rupture. I was settled on this doctor and only left him because during the first trimester, I decided it would be better for me to move states, set up my life, and have the baby in Georgia.

When I arrived in Georgia from New Jersey, I had already identified an OB office and a doctor that had amazing reviews, who had also graduated from my alma mater. When I reached out to see if I could become his patient, the office took about a week to come back to me and say no. He didn't want to take any new patients at the time, which was understandable. There were about 12 other OBs at that office so I asked for a few other OBs specifically by name; it took the office almost 2 weeks to come back and tell me no for each doctor. Ultimately, they attempted to assign a doctor to me. The doctor they wanted to assign had terrible Google reviews which is why I had not asked for her. The office administrator in charge of transfers was rather rude to me on the phone, and left me on hold indefinitely on more than one occasion. She had initially told me that past 17 weeks pregnant, I would not be able to transfer into their practice. Meanwhile, she was increasing my pregnancy "age", by taking such a long time to let me know if I could become a patient of the doctors I was selecting, only to turn around and tell me no each time. I was very disheartened. The move to Georgia had been overwhelming, even though I went to high school there and had some family there. I was growing more and more alarmed that I did not have a doctor in place for almost a month.

By this point pregnancy hormones were in full effect so every problem seemed like the end of the world to me. I knew what hospital I wanted to deliver with so I was working backwards, from their website, to find doctors to interview. *This was a major key.* I wanted to deliver at a facility that could handle any type of possible emergency and that would respect my birth plan for my child. The hospital I chose in Atlanta is known as the "baby factory", and I knew that even though I was a bit of a 50-year-old unicorn, I was not the first one they had ever seen, which was very important to me. After my poor experience with the first OB group, I then interviewed another doctor at a different OB group because she also had great reviews. After meeting with her, it seemed like she was close to retirement. She just seemed a bit low energy like she was over the demands of being an on call OB which is understandable, but not ideal for the experience I wished to have. I just didn't feel 100% secure with her, so I kept looking. In the end I selected an OB from a third large OB group in the city, who also attended the same school that I did, who is close in age to me. We had actually had the same chemistry professors in college, and she was really energetic, awesome and supportive. She was also clear about the plan and how we should proceed. She felt that we should continue with the same plan my male OB from New Jersey set out, and that's what we did.

My Georgia OB told me that I would also have to have a maternal-fetal medicine doctor (MFM) which I knew because I also had a maternal-fetal medicine doctor in New Jersey. Both of my MFMs were awesome and had so much experience, knowledge and stories to share. With my pregnancy being so-called high risk, I saw them very often which meant I got to see my baby a lot during the growing process. My maternal-fetal medicine doctor in New Jersey was a beautiful and chic woman in her late thirties. She told me about all the different experiences she had had with more mature moms. She had even delivered a baby to a woman who was 67 years old. That woman had a boyfriend who was in his 40s. They loved each other so much that they wanted to have a child together. Obviously, they used a donor egg. She said the woman was in great shape and the delivery was uneventful. My maternal-fetal medicine doctor in Atlanta had at least 30 decades of experience. He was amazing and just so thorough in each of our ultrasound appointments looking for every possible thing that could be an issue like gestational diabetes and preeclampsia. He explained everything he was visualizing in each ultrasound. I had a wonderful team which helped aid my peace of mind. I made sure to ask every question and do all the research on each physician which honestly, can take a long time but is worth it in the end because everyone on the team is dialed in for your best interest. I think the most important questions you want to ask are: have they worked with someone your age? What sort of problems or issues are they going to be keeping an eye out for? And what is their plan of action because you want to make sure that it matches your own. If you are dreaming of a VBAC and they are adamantly advising a C-section, you have to get on the same page. You want to know if this is the person that's going to be delivering your baby or might it be someone else on their team? If you are older with an IVF pregnancy, they may want to do a C-section in which case your OB can schedule the surgery when it is convenient for you both, and you have assurance of who will deliver. But if you deliver vaginally, your OB may not be on call. I wanted to avoid this at all costs. It's a little nerve wracking getting to the hospital to deliver and then having to do it with some doctor that you've never even met. Black women have the highest incidence of maternal death and I wanted to be 100 percent sure of who was doing my delivery. You run your team and hopefully your maternal-fetal medicine doctor and your OB are a part of the same network because it makes things much easier.

It's always surprising for people to hear stories like this of women in their 50s and 60s having babies. I even read a story about a woman in India who delivered a baby at 72 because that was the only way that she and her husband could get the husband's inheritance from his father. In order for his father's money to land with him, it was contingent upon him having a child. So they went to an IVF clinic and the wife, at 71 years old, got pregnant. After reading all of these stories, my mindset became, well I'm not the first, and I certainly won't be the last. Mindset is everything. After I was well into the process, these kinds of stories just kept coming up in my social media feeds. I saw reminders about how Janet Jackson got pregnant and delivered her son at 50. I saw Brigitte Nielsen get pregnant at age 54. Whether they were doing it naturally or through IVF was immaterial to me because I have friends in their 30s who for whatever reason were having to turn to IVF and donor eggs as well as sperm, so there was no shame or distinction in IVF, in my estimation.

Supplements, Acupuncture and Exercise – PRE-IVF

From my failed egg freezing days I had become familiar with the benefits of acupuncture and all of the various Chinese herbs and supplements that one could take to either boost fertility or just enhance their overall health. I come from a family of people who eat very healthily. My father was a chef and heavily into juicing, fasting and Chinese herbs. My mom always made us eat vegetables and drink water, no sugar sodas allowed when we were growing up. My stepmother is a raw vegan. Both of my grandmothers ate primarily vegetables and beans with the occasional roast protein. I have never eaten pork in my life, and have been heavy on organic food for the last 8 years. So I've mostly been on a trajectory of health leading up to getting pregnant, minus some alcohol drinking which I completely dropped when I made the decision to take this journey. I was eating for fertility which mainly meant fresh fruits and vegetables, lots of cold pressed beet juice and green juice, lean meats, fish and organic chicken. I was also eating a ton of fresh pineapple which has bromelain in it, which the Google machine says is supposed to aid in embryo implantation.

I knew that I was in perimenopause or menopause, so I began taking omega 3 as a liquid, which Google said was to support my heart health. I knew that I would need a strong heart to support the extra task of growing a baby. I took

CoQ10 as a liquid to counterbalance any oxidative stress on my cells. I wanted the cells to replicate as well as possible, especially when the embryo was transferred. I started taking liquid chlorophyll to help detox my body and counteract any inflammation. I was also taking magnesium which is touted to reduce risk of preeclampsia and fetal growth restriction. I was already taking vitamin B, vitamin D, and zinc because I wanted to stay covid free, which was important because you cannot be sick running in and out of these clinics and doctor's offices. I was of course taking prenatals. I tried several brands that I was buying from Amazon, and they weren't doing anything for me. The doctor ended up giving me a prescription prenatal called Westab Plus that I am still taking today. It was huge, like a big horse pill, but I could definitely feel a difference in my energy levels after I began taking it. I was also taking the liquid iron and the Cat's Claw to get my CBC readouts more in the normal range, that I mentioned before. I was drinking turmeric tea as an anti-inflammatory, as well as dandelion tea as a detox a couple times a week. Wooosa!

Taking all these supplements every day takes me about 20 minutes. I always laugh and say it is very labor intensive. My mother was curious about my reasoning for taking so many supplements, but I still take most of them to this day as part of my youthful longevity journey. I don't take all of them *every day* because my nausea can't handle so many supplements at once. In addition to taking supplements, I was drinking electrolyte water, consisting of the reverse osmosis filtration system water from my countertop machine with organic lime juice squeezed in it and sometimes a pinch of sea salt.

I had not done any acupuncture since living in LA four years prior. Covid pretty much stopped everything for me. But I wanted to cover all of my bases with this procedure so I started acupuncture about two months before we did the frozen embryo transfer. Acupuncture is amazing for pretty much anything that ails you so when I was looking for an acupuncturist, I made sure to look for a fertility acupuncturist. I got really specific about that and I wanted someone from the culture who knew exactly what they were doing. I found a great place near me with a woman practitioner who also had fertility issues. She shared with me that acupuncture helped her to have her son. So I felt like I was in great hands. We did a mixture of acupuncture and cupping to get the blood flowing in my body and to be less stagnant. She did not give me or recommend any Chinese herbs, which was probably for the best because I was already taking eight million supplements as it was.

As it relates to working out, I'm not a big gym person, but I love to dance, so I did a lot of stretching and movement and every now and then I would get on the elliptical. But that's about it, I didn't go crazy because I wasn't trying to lose weight. Again, I was just working to get my blood flow up to snuff, because my job and my life tends to be very sedentary. With exercise, I tend to stick to whatever exercise that I can commit to without having to leave my home. I knew that I was trying to build a nice fluffy environment for my embryo to implant. So I just focused on activities to make the blood flow, and make me flush with health like dancing, stretching, pilates mat, etc. I watched a lot of YouTube along this journey and I saw many women on YouTube who are total athletes train very hard and were able to keep up their routines until the middle of their pregnancy, and good on them, but that has never been my ministry. But I also do get that if you are a little bit overweight, then you do actually want to lose weight and get to a healthy size before you become pregnant and gain more weight. This is totally understandable. I didn't really gain weight during my pregnancy. Any weight that I gained was literally just the baby and fluid. I might have gained 20 pounds the whole pregnancy. And in fact, on the bottom, I looked smaller. The baby ended up eating my prized booty and hips. It made me laugh the entire pregnancy, it was so completely unexpected.

Detox and Immunology

On the TTC (trying to conceive) internet message boards we talk a lot about our supplements, injections, and hormones, but we don't talk enough about detoxing our bodies, and we certainly don't talk enough about the rise in immune issues which are causing IVF cycles to fail in many women. I had done a deep dive on all the toxins we use in our cosmetics, nail glues, eyelash glues and parabens in lotions that can cause a heavy toxic load on our reproductive systems, to say nothing of the processed and non organic food. There is a "dirty dozen" list published each year that lists the fruits and vegetables that have been found to have the most pesticides on them, and these are the ones that you want to make sure that you purchase organically. Although the offenders on the list change each year as you will find when you Google them, you can pretty much always find strawberries, greens (mustard, kale, collard), apples, peaches, celery and tomatoes on this list. After prioritizing the organic items on my grocery list, I ruthlessly went through my house throwing out dishwashing liquids, bathroom cleaners, many of my prized beauty products and got myself on a regimen of minimalism. I was only using olive oil as a moisturizer, I was only using basic soaps and cleaners for the house. I stopped relaxing my hair. I drank reverse osmosis filtered water. I believe that some of these changes were a big help for me. At any rate, they could not hurt.

There is an NYC based fertility influencer named Tanika, she goes by Simply Tanika. She is a few years older than me and fell pregnant a few months before I did. She was documenting her journey on YouTube. She had several failed frozen embryo transfers but was so regimented with all of her diet and supplements that the doctor had a hard time pinpointing why her uterus was not accepting them. After several attempts her IVF doctor sent her to a reproductive immunologist (RI) to do a workup and get to the bottom of things. She generously recorded her phone call with the RI for YouTube and I'll never forget that one of several medicines they put her on was hydroxychloroquine. My eyebrows raised all the way up because hydroxychloroquine had become such a demonized medicine for the mainstream media during the covid pandemic. It was a shame because it's just a medicine that is used to treat malaria and some autoimmune diseases. I remember being very interested in her prescribed protocol to quiet down her autoimmune issues that were becoming an obstacle to pregnancy, and watching to see if the RI's treatment for her would work. It did work. She has a son that is 4 months older than my own. I made a note that if I had the same issue where my uterus was repeatedly rejecting embryos that I would go to see a reproductive immunologist as well. There has been an alarming rise in autoimmune diseases in Western countries within the last 4 decades. No one really seems to be able to pinpoint what is causing this other than the environment and pollutants. Either way, it is something to work against by detoxifying our lives as much as possible and keeping the phone number of a good immunologist in our contact lists.

Mindset Of A Mom

I think that working through the traditional adoption classes, paperwork and background checks made me see myself more and more as a mother in my mind long before I ever began the journey to being pregnant. Viewing myself as a "mom" in my mind, I believe helped me become a vibrational match to the outcome I desired. I know this sounds woo-woo, but ultimately, everything we see is made up of the same energetic "stuff", and that "stuff" that creates exists at different frequencies which allows it to show up in different forms. For example, water can be ice, liquid or steam. It shows up in three distinct forms, but is the same thing at a source level in each form. So being a "mom" in my mind, buying items for my baby as though he was already here and planning for him as though he was here I believe, allowed a more frictionless way for him to actually arrive. I find this to be hard work mentally, to constantly be trying to live from the end, which simply means living in my desired result mentally, until it is manifested outwardly. As Yeshua says, in Mark 11:24, "therefore I say unto you, what things soever ye desire, when ye pray, believe that ye receive them, and ye shall have them", which led me to believe that the receiving is actually rooted in the believing and acting as if, with a bit of a time delay since we are here on earth and not in heaven. I had to stop giving attention to the very real problems I had, which were daily staring me in my face. I had no eggs left, and I was 49 and single. But every day I would focus on my desired result, which was a child in my arms. I had a mental picture of it. I saw myself in my kitchen with a little toddler dressed in a snowsuit. I would pick him up, sit him on the counter, and help him put on his mittens. It's a very weird and specific picture. But that was my mental picture, and it would make me feel warm and fuzzy when I thought about it like it was my real life and I was already doing it.

About 10 months before I got pregnant, I was shopping for a gift for my niece in the toy section of Target and I saw a little baby doll. It was a little boy baby doll in a onesie and I had the urge to purchase him for myself so I did. Maybe I bought him with the thought of practicing changing diapers and putting on and taking off clothes. I have seen so many shows where students and kids have to practice maintaining dolls as real babies 24/7 for a period of time to discourage them from having children prematurely, so it did cross my mind that I need to get my expectations level set of what having a baby would be like. At this point I was deep in the traditional adoption process as well, and had just met with that young expectant mother. Practicing living from the end was becoming more and more important to me, so I would hang out with the doll while watching Netflix. I would pack the doll when I would drive an hour and half south to visit my mom in Atlantic City. She thought I was nuts. Every time I would come to see her, I would have this baby doll with me and she would say, "you brought that doll again?" And I'd say, "yeah" as she would just shake her head and I would laugh. I was working on my believing.

I also had set up the bassinet in my room that I had purchased from the time when I thought that adoption was imminent. After that fell through, for some reason I just never took the bassinet down. It was bedside in my room for the better part of a year. And I would set the baby doll in there when I wasn't dealing with it which honestly was most of the time. I was working 16 to 18 hour days so I didn't have a lot of time to play with the baby doll but it was just there, hanging out in the background, throughout that whole year.

Back in 2021 I drew a stick drawing of a ranch house in Georgia with me as the stick person standing in front of the house holding another little stick person. Today I live in a ranch house in Georgia with a little person. Day after day, I looked at that stick drawing for probably one and a half years. I started that meditation long before I even knew that embryo adoption was a thing. That meditation was really about me adopting a baby or so I thought. I also had an auto suggestion recording in my phone. I would play inspirational songs or gospel songs that I liked in the background and then I would talk about my life in present day terms, but describing what I wanted to see. I would talk as though I already had the child. I had already moved and I would describe these things in my voice. And then I would just play the recording back to myself at random times during the day to stimulate my subconscious into believing it. I really do believe that mindset is more than 50% of what we get in life. Historically I tend to be conservatively negative, so as not to be disappointed, and I have to work harder to prime myself to be a match to the wonderful things in life that I say that I want. It's taken me 50 years to figure this out, but better late than never.

I'm a Christian, and I pray daily. I make sure to pray active prayers. I give my angels assignments. I bind and I loose in the spirit realm (Matthew 18:18). I pray that no weapon formed against me shall prosper (Isaiah 54:17). I don't think that it's paranoid to think that there are folks who don't wish for your success in every area of your life. Not everyone is as good a person as you are, Dear Reader. And so I do pray that any prayers that are activated against me are nullified, cut off, frustrated and foiled. I believe that the prayers of my grandmothers over me are still active as well. And then I work as hard as I can to believe the best. Like I said, this type of mental and spiritual work is definitely heavy lifting, but I find that when I do it, it definitely puts me in a higher mood or frequency. And I believe it makes me more able to receive the goodness that exists.

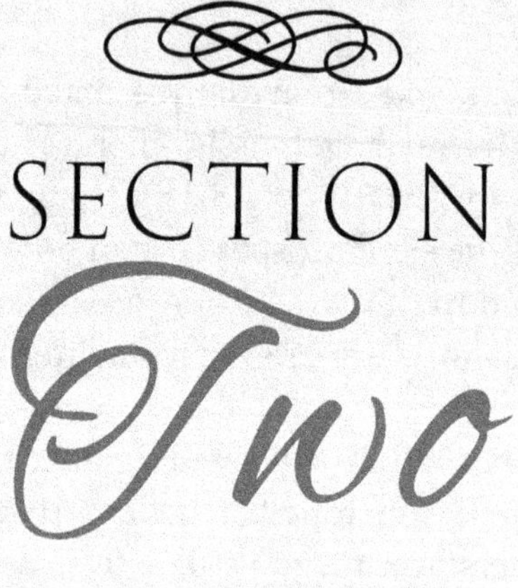

SECTION *Two*

IVF AND PREGNANCY

IVF

I would say one of the best things about my IVF experience was doing the prep month of estrogen and progesterone in order to trigger a period and shedding of the lining of the uterus. It had been about a year since I had a period on my own and when your hormones are shifting like that in a slow, gradual way, you don't really recognize what's missing. But with the addition of the estrogen and the progesterone, I began to feel like my old self. I felt a little less aggressive, and a little more bouncy, which again, no one would really describe me as bouncy, but that's how I felt. In taking those hormones during that prep month I realized that I should have been supporting my body with some sort of hormonal boosting or stimulating once I went into menopause, but I did not know what I should be taking. I knew I didn't want to take synthetics for the rest of my life, so I had just let it go, not knowing why I was feeling off. It was something I knew that I needed to look into and address after the baby was born.

After our prep month we were on to the frozen embryo transfer. This was exciting for me because I had never gotten this far in anything I had tried previously. I had never come this close to a possible victory in the entire decade of trying to become a mother by whatever means necessary. I worked on trying to get as much sleep and rest as I possibly could. I didn't want any additional stress on my body. As it happened, I had been laid off of my job a few weeks before my transfer, and while it was distressing from a financial point of view, it was the best thing that could have happened to me. I know, I've mentioned the high stress nature of the job several times already and I was very worried that it was going to affect the pregnancy. With being laid off in this way, that job was not allowed to touch my pregnancy and I feel like that was important for me and my son. I was getting rest. I was working on my mind. I was eating well. I was going to acupuncture a few times a week and I was taking the hormones. For the second month of hormones leading up to the frozen embryo transfer, we added in the progesterone shot in the behind. It was interesting and relatively painful, shooting myself in the booty. But I was happy even to do that because again, it was an indication that I was getting closer to my dream. As I was taking the estrogen and progesterone shots, I was also going into the clinic for measurements of the uterus lining to make sure that it was growing nice and fluffy so that the embryo could implant. Some women will do an acupuncture session immediately before the transfer. For instance, they'll go to their acupuncturist for a session, leave that office, go to their IVF clinic for the transfer, leave the IVF clinic, go back to the acupuncture office for another session and then go home. But my acupuncturist is highly sought after and very busy. She had no openings on the day of my transfer. Also when I asked her about doing that, she indicated that she thought it was unnecessary and that acupuncture doesn't work that way. She said it was a cumulative effect from getting treatment over time. So we ended up doing a session 3 days before the transfer and then 2 days after.

The actual day of the frozen embryo transfer was the briefest of all of the appointments that I had with my clinic. I don't know quite what I expected; perhaps, more fanfare. I went in and sat in the waiting room for about 10 minutes, then was ushered back into the transfer suite. The nurse came in with the doctor and the embryologist. She handed him the embryo, he delivered it into my uterus via a super small catheter which took about a minute. We had some chat afterward which consisted mainly of instructions and well wishes, and then I left. I would say the whole visit may have taken about 30 minutes. When he implanted the embryo I didn't really feel anything at first. I went to my car and ate some more pineapple and recorded a vlog as I had been vlogging the entire experience for YouTube. Then I laid in the back of the car, and I put my legs in the air. I laid like that for about 40 minutes before undertaking the hour's drive back to my side of town. After that I went to a park that has a lake and I walked around the lake just to get the blood flowing to my uterus. The lake is next door to a zoo and there was a big banner depicting a lioness and a baby lion cub. The lion has significance for me because Yeshua is the Lion of Judah. The other significance obviously being the mama/baby symbolism in the picture. I had never noticed that banner before at the lake, so I took that as a special hug from The Most High. I finished my walk, went home and ordered my favorite take-out.

On that day and in the days to follow, I did feel tickling or implantation tugging. There was a feeling of pressure in my uterus when I would lay flat on my back. But so many women report that they feel nothing after transferring that you begin to question any feeling you do have. You wonder if you are just fooling yourself because how could you possibly feel anything with an embryo that small? I transferred a day 5 embryo which is pretty mature in the embryo creation process so it wasn't nothing, but still I had a nagging voice in the back of my mind questioning these sensations that I arduously tried to ignore. I went to a Jill Scott concert the next week, and it was a very tight venue so you couldn't really stand up and dance around. I was dancing and shaking my hips in my chair. I then got a little nervous, thinking I needed to calm down with all of the hip wiggling because I didn't want to knock the embryo loose. This was probably nonsense but there were all sorts of thoughts flying around.

I had another acupuncture session 2 days later, and another one a week after. My wait time for blood work was 9 days since I implanted a day 5 embryo. I decided not to do a home test in the 9 days following the transfer because I didn't want to see something that would get me started on a negative tailspin of thoughts. I knew how vitally important it was to think the right thoughts during this time. After I went to the clinic to do the first round of beta (Beta-hCG) blood work post transfer, as I was still waiting for the yay or nay phone call, I did take a cheap $5 home pregnancy test because I figured, it couldn't hurt at that point and would prepare me for the call if it was bad news. But, the cheap test only showed 1 line! My heart dropped down into my socks. I was so crestfallen. I sat down at my computer and just started responding to emails like crazy in an attempt to get a hold of myself and not spiral down into the abyss. The clinic had not called me yet but my mind was exploding with every random, terrible thought possible. This was precisely the reason why I had abstained from doing any home tests during those 9 days. About an hour after taking the cheap test, I got a call from the clinic with the news I had been waiting ten years to hear! I was pregnant! I was in shock. I wanted to repeat the experience of receiving the news again, so I went out to CVS and got a proper First Response test, and that had a bright, resounding, second "pregnant" line on it, so it just goes to show you that sometimes the tests, especially those cheap ones can play games with you.

My first beta blood work came back at 238. My second beta bloodwork came back at 938, which was more than the doubling of the number that they look for to indicate that things are progressing. So then, we could be confident that I was well and truly pregnant and had both feet firmly planted in the midst of my new adventure!

Pregnancy Symptoms

Once I knew I was pregnant, I dropped all supplements except for my prenatal, vitamin B, vitamin D, magnesium and liquid iron. I didn't want anything to interfere with the baby's development. My plan was just to eat and drink properly and let him grow.

Typically, I'm not a person who eats much. As a child, I didn't like eating, I thought it was basically a waste of time. I still am of that mindset, really. It takes so much time to prepare the food, eat it, wash up the dishes and the kitchen and then you are expected to do that 3 times a day?! Normally, I don't eat what people would call a proper breakfast, but I do have fruit or a slice of bread to take my vitamins and supplements. I rarely eat lunch unless I am stress-eating last night's leftovers, but I do eat a hearty dinner and I do like to snack. Obviously, I had to throw all of that out the window. By week 3 I was ravenous, so I would get up and eat whatever was available. I was definitely having lunch and I wasn't denying myself either because I knew that my body needed all the energy I could get for the cells of the embryo to grow and proliferate. I began eating breakfast foods like scrambled eggs for as long as I could stand the smell, and then I switched to boiled eggs and toast. I was still obsessed with my cold press juices. I was having those every day. I would have spinach croissants for lunch. And then for dinner, I was having a lot of lamb, fish and organic chicken which I was eating before.

Regarding my sleep habits, I am a person who needs plenty of sleep but does not like to sleep. I'm like a child in that way. I could sleep twelve hours a day if I didn't have work and life obligations, but I always wake up chastising myself about all I haven't gotten done so I try to keep the sleeping to 6 to 8 hours when I'm not pregnant. I found that during pregnancy, I was desperately sleepy. Literally, I was so sleepy, I could cry. I'd never felt this type of sleepiness before, and it was a little frustrating because it felt like I couldn't get any work accomplished.

I also found that because of the hormones that I was taking in that first trimester, I was out of breath a lot. Even trying to stand up and cook in the kitchen was a challenge. I would have to bring a stool in and sit down because I was weirdly out of breath. That went away after I stopped taking the progesterone and estrogen. I also found that I was fighting a little bit of depression in that first trimester and I know that was hormonal as well. It was such a dichotomy to be so happy and overjoyed about finally being pregnant, but then to feel this weird tinge of depression at the same time, because you have no idea where it's coming from. Once I sensed it and was able to name it, I just kept an eye on it, but I didn't notice it anymore after I was able to get off of the hormones in the second trimester. The depression went away completely.

The other thing I noticed was how keen my nose became and how everything smelled terrible. At the time, I lived in a relatively new apartment building. The building was maybe 4 years old at the time that I became pregnant. After I became pregnant, I could smell the pipes, or at least I thought I could smell the pipes, and I became such a nuisance to the poor maintenance team of the building. I kept putting in complaints that the pipes were backed up. They kept coming to my apartment to snake the shower and kitchen sink pipes. Then they would pour deodorizer down them. I think they did this three times and I would still complain. I know they were sick of me! I felt as though I could even smell it coming through the washing machine! When I had visitors come to my apartment I'd complain and ask them could they smell anything? Everyone said no. I finally realized that it was being pregnant that was playing tricks on my nose, once I realized everything smelled bad everywhere I went. I had a supersonic nose whereas everyone else had a normal one. I also couldn't taste food in the same way that I tasted it pre-pregnancy. It was like my taste buds were diminished in some way, perhaps to offset my nose's new capabilities! I went to Miami in week 6 and I went to some wonderful, fabulous places to eat but couldn't really taste the flavor of any of the food which was a shame. But all of it was in service of the overriding goal, so even though it was inconvenient, it was the tiniest price to pay.

Morning sickness was not really an issue for me. I experienced nausea at random times. It was never in the morning, but always in the middle of the afternoon, in the heat of the summer, and twice I got sick while driving. So embarrassing, to be driving while throwing up in a plastic bag, or puking my guts out in a mall parking lot as cars drive past. But for the few times I experienced sickness, it was nothing compared to the women who are sick every day of their pregnancy of which there are many.

Village

No matter what time of life you have your baby, and no matter how capable a mother you are, your village is vital. As a single mother by choice or default, depending on how you look at it, I knew I would need as much village support as I could get. Most of my friends had already had their babies. I have some friends who are actually new grandparents, as I am just getting started welcoming my first child so I had to take inventory. I was living in New Jersey and I have family up-and-down the East Coast. Initially, I planned to stay in New Jersey, but throughout the first trimester, it became clearer and clearer to me that I needed to move in order to set up our lives`in a way that made the most sense and with the closest support available to us. My mother came to my apartment and literally packed all of my boxes and I moved south in the 12th week of my pregnancy.

I had to consider the notion that some of my relatives may not have agreed with what I was doing. As it happened, some relatives stopped speaking to me abruptly. I didn't know what the issue was. Even when I moved, some of the reactions from my friends were confusing and not ideal while the reactions of other friends were so amazing. You never know who is going to be an angel for you. It is easy to assume bad intent when you think people are treating you poorly, but it's not always the truth. One thing I learned about being pregnant is that it is the one time when you are super clear about your mission. Whatever other people's reactions may be, are for them to deal with. I would not waste time sussing out the motivations behind certain behaviors that may have had nothing to do with me. Also, pregnancy means your hormones are heightened and so are your moods. Your anger is more angry. Your happiness is more happy. Your sadness and disappointment are intensified. I had to bear that in mind to try to modulate my responses in certain situations. I didn't always navigate that successfully but I managed to finally understand that the right people, who were supposed to be a part of my child's life would show up. They did show up and have been showing up for me, which at the end of the day is all that matters. Despite the ups and downs, I find that every day, the decision to move was the right one and has been so central to my peace of mind and by extension, to my son's happiness.

Pregnancy is also probably the best time to start interviewing people for child care services, whether that's someone coming into your home or whether that's you taking the baby to daycare which I know can be very scary for parents. Or, it could even mean lining up a family member or friend to watch the baby, as well as having your backup babysitters for nighttime going out. I know a woman who got her child into a Montessori day care when she was early in her second trimester. Meanwhile, I didn't even think about anyone outside of my family, watching my son until now and he is 6 months old. I never go anywhere. When you think about it, especially considering how much I used to socialize, it is kind of crazy, but I was so happy to be in the house with him that I really had no desire to go outside. That's one of the primary benefits of waiting until 50 to have a baby. I had already gone to all the parties, taken so many trips, walked some red carpets, been to the nightclubs and all the concerts. By the time my son came, no one could make me feel like I was missing anything.

As humans though, we do need, not necessarily balance, but perhaps, variety. Even I know it can't be all kids, all the time. I definitely want to be a parent who remains myself, so that I don't have to start over, creating a life when my child starts to pull away to create his own life with his own friends. Some women need a lot more "me time" and time with friends to feel like themselves. If this is you, and you don't have family nearby to watch the baby, then second trimester is a good time to be doing those interviews and background checks. If you use a home care or sitter website that offers you a wide range of choices for caregivers, you want to narrow down your list to 5 to 10 people and do your interviews at a coffee shop so they don't have to come to your home before you've actually done any type of background check. Be very clear about what the rate of pay will be in your advertisement on the site, and don't negotiate. The people willing to work for your rate of pay will be the people you will be choosing from. Be very clear about your expectations. If you are looking for someone to do more than just feed the baby, and play a little bit, then set that expectation. If you want someone to wash dishes and do some laundry, be explicit about that. If you want someone keeping a schedule of reading and teaching and playing with Montessori type toys, displaying flash cards and things of this nature then put all of that into the advertisement. If you won't allow any screens around the baby, put that in the advertisement as well. Some people who will apply will just be looking for an easy gig of feeding and sleeping the baby and you want to weed those folks out from the beginning.

Time Management

No one manages time. We manage activities, which means we need to prioritize well. I was fortunate during my pregnancy. I had just been laid off so I had time to get set up relatively stress-free. I had time to sleep more, even while I was still working on my own business. But if a woman already has a family, has a demanding job and is pregnant, that woman is going to feel like she is in a pressure cooker. Like most expecting mamas, I was on websites like What to Expect and saw that other women were saying that you want to do all of your house prep and purchase the things you'll need in trimester two. Foolishly, I did not do that because I was still in the process of just setting up the house from the cross state move. I also spent most of my second trimester, after my 50th birthday, planning my baby shower. I had not thrown myself a party for 11 years and I saw the shower as a real opportunity to celebrate, so planning took over my life for the better part of two months. I also wanted to wait until after the shower to take inventory of what had and had not come in so I could purchase the remainder of the shower registry and then dig into setting up the nest. With all of that going on, I didn't even really focus on what I needed for the baby until the beginning of trimester 3, which I would say was a mistake. I should have pressed harder in trimester 2. As the baby got heavier, my ability to stand for long periods diminished. My child loves to kick even until this day, and obviously, while in utero, the more he kicked, the less I slept at night and the more tired I was during the day. I found myself really pressed and rushing to get the last minute items I needed. For instance, I purchased a hospital bedside table for my bedroom so that I could set up the computer for work and not have to put it on my lap. I bought a grabber stick so that I didn't have to do too much twisting to reach and pick things up post-surgery; I could just use this long pincher stick. I purchased toilet rails to help me get up-and-down from my very low seated toilet so I wouldn't have to grab at the walls to sit and stand. I bought a tiny fridge for my bedside table and a diaper cart for bedside as well. I set up everything so that I had as little inconvenience as possible post-surgery. I made gallons of homemade chicken soup and froze them because I knew I wouldn't be cooking those first weeks back home. But I could have been doing that in second trimester, too since they were going to be frozen anyway. Now of course, the final cleaning of the house you really can't do until third trimester and you may even have to hire somebody to do that because it's not like you can really get down to the baseboards when you're as big as the house itself. But for the women who do, props to them!

Being Practical, Leaving A Legacy and Longevity

So this is the part where a lot of people want to scold you about having a baby as a mature person or a person in midlife because they feel like it's a selfish act. When I was a child, my village consisted primarily of my grandparents. My mother would get us out of school for the summer and before we knew it we would be packed up in the car on the way to be dropped off at her mother's house where we would stay for most of the summer. Then, that grandmother would put us on a bus and send us to the other grandmother's house, where we would stay for a few weeks. And at the end of the summer, we would go back home for school. My mother had every summer off and my grandmothers loved having us. I was unusually close with both of them. My father's mother did not pass until she was 87 and I was 40 years old and my mother's mother did not pass until she was 92 and I was 46. You have to bear in mind also that these people also smoked unfiltered cigarettes for over half of their lives! They grew up in tobacco country after all. They had exceptionally robust vigor. So it's a foreign concept for me to think that my child won't have a full life with me. My father passed away when he was 74 and I was 45 and I still have a living parent today, my mother, who is 78.

All of that is immaterial though, because whether I've had a baby at 30 or 40 or 50, I know that it's essential to leave your child set up for whenever it is that you do take your exit. So I went ahead and bought a few life insurance policies. I created an explicit will and had it notarized. I went ahead and made a plan for guardianship, and I set up his trust and custodial investment accounts. Doing these things made me feel more secure for him. What's more ironic is that if I'd had my child at 30, I probably wouldn't have done any of those things, or I would have done those things after he'd already arrived. At that point in time, I just wasn't very dialed in with all of my finances and the business aspects of my life. I'm way more responsible now than I was 10 or 20 years ago, so I definitely feel as though my son is benefitting from my decades of experience. Having planned and paid for a few funerals now, I have a much different perspective on what those who are left behind will need should they be faced with a sad situation, such as the loss of a parent. But my intention is to live long and strong. With long life I pray God will satisfy me and show me his salvation (Psalm 91:16).

I run a brand called Youthful Longevity, which is dedicated to the celebration of maturing with vigor and style. My supplement routine, my dancing routine, and my eating are all designed to take me from 50 to 100 years old and beyond. The Pew Research Center says that the U.S. centenarian population will quadruple in the next 30 years which makes sense.[2] Most of us don't smoke like our parents and grandparents did. Many of us don't drink. We wear seat belts and eat organically with as few pesticides as possible. I have made a study, researching centenarians to find out what is the secret to their longevity. Their routines vary widely to be honest,

2   https://www.pewresearch.org/short-reads/2024/01/09/us-centenarian-population-is-projected-to-quadruple-over-the-next-30-years/

but they almost all talk about the positioning of their hearts, not holding grudges, keeping life simple, and eating relatively healthily. One gentleman though, Vincent Dransfield, has a part of his routine that is my favorite secret. He drinks Ovaltine every day. He is 110 years old as of 2024, lives on his own in New Jersey, drives himself around, and he credits some of his longevity to having worked on the dairy farms of New Jersey as a youngster and having that good milk to drink during the Great Depression. He believes it strengthened his bones and immunity and gave him a good start in life. He drinks Ovaltine every day, and is such a champion of it that everyone who attended his 100th birthday party ten years ago drank a glass of Ovaltine as well. I can't tell you how fast I went out and bought some Ovaltine after reading that story. Now I enjoy a chocolate glass of goodness every day. Aside from all of the normal vitamins in Ovaltine, it also has a good supply of copper which according to Google, is known to help the body make red blood cells and keep the immune system healthy.

You Are Not Just You Anymore

"It's not just you anymore". People will say that to you very often during pregnancy, but one thing I was not prepared for was having a hard time accessing my own baseline "vibe". We all have a baseline energy that we show up in if we are not stressed or in conflict. I still felt like myself, but definitely different. The baby had his own distinct vibe and it was mixing with mine. So when I would go to pray and meditate, I would have a hard time feeling how I used to feel before. It's not that the baby had any type of negative vibe or feeling, but his energy was so strong that it just made me keep noticing him. Because my meditating felt so different now, I found myself doing it less. I began drifting on my early morning personal development work. It was very hard to concentrate sometimes. That was one of the things that I wish I had known ahead of time and maybe, I could have put some fail safes in action so that I wouldn't have had as much drift, but I was completely distracted by the time we got to the middle of the pregnancy. It wasn't until he "moved out" of my belly that I really felt like myself again.

Planning For Maternity Leave

At this point I was working for myself scaling a small business. Many of the menial tasks I was performing, and then I had two virtual assistants helping me as well. I intended to front-load a good bit of my work so that I could at least have a few weeks to not have to open the computer after the baby was born. I did not do as great a job of that as I should have done. I was able to not check in for about a week and a half, and then I did start having to hop on my laptop and do some work here and there. My son was born in November and I was at the last minute putting together a Black Friday promotion so I didn't really plan my leave well. If I were to do it over again, I would start really planning for that maternity leave, meaning setting up automations for sales letters and planning my ads at least 3 months before the birth of the baby. In the back of my mind, I thought I would be able to manage working on the computer and trying to think through sales plans and deal with the baby at the same time. Foolishness. I erroneously thought the baby would sleep a lot more than he did and that I would not have 10 million other things to do while he was sleeping like pumping breastmilk and feeding myself! My poor planning meant that the business suffered in ways it didn't have to if I had planned better from the beginning.

I also would say that if you can come up with any other kind of other side hustle before the baby arrives like finally selling your famous cupcakes in the neighborhood, or finally selling your business excel spreadsheets with the formulas preloaded, it is a good thing. Any kind of business you control is great because if you decide you just don't have the desire to go back to work after the baby arrives, then you already have a head start on an income replacement and perhaps a little less pushback from your partner if you decide that you want to stay home. Negotiating with your employer about when you're going to come back and trying to find ways to extend maternity leave just becomes extra stress while you are getting adjusted at home and trying to heal. Even moreso, if you were previously in a job you hated. I see this a lot on the pregnancy message boards that I belong to. Women did not want to go back to their incredibly stressful jobs. Then adding the anxiety of taking a child to a daycare on top of that was really crippling for some women. Even though I was not in that particular situation, I wish I had pressed a little harder to stack up my work for more weeks in advance. I ended up taking time away from my baby to do work. It would have been nice to have all that time for the baby and not to have had to look at the business at all.

Doulas and C-Sections

I went back and forth about whether or not I should have a doula with me in surgery. A few people that I floated the idea by swiveled their necks at me and said "why?!", when I mentioned that I was thinking about hiring one. The main reason for me was that I wanted someone who could advocate for me assertively, yet pleasantly, while I was incapacitated and cut open. Because I don't have a partner in this journey, I feel as though the most crucial part where you do need support is in the actual birthing. You're dealing with a lot of professional staff, doctors and nurses who are moving quickly. And while I had done a great deal of background research to make sure that I had the right people on my team, I still wanted to make sure that someone could go with the baby if he had to go to the neonatal unit or if anything went wrong.

I wanted to make sure that someone was with the baby for every step of the way post-birth, and that my birth plan for him was respected. This way we both had an advocate.

While I didn't need anyone to help me breathe and push because I didn't experience labor, it was nice to have someone there while I was getting my epidural. It was nice to have someone keep eyes on the baby while I was being sewn up. I suppose this role could have also been a family member, but a family member is not going to handle the stress of the moment in quite the same way, or have as much birthing information as a professional doula. My entire goal was to reduce my stress. Now, I wasn't entirely successful in this mission, but I tried. I also wanted to have the doula come to the house to help me after my hospital stay. I anticipated going home alone and having the occasional visitor stop by with food. As it happened, my aunt and my cousin were there with me every step of the way. My cousin stayed in my guest room for a week afterwards and my aunt was there all the time as well, so baby and I were in no way alone at any time. But I still hired the doula for two days afterward to come in and help with the baby, while I was trying to rest, work and just get back to normal. Obviously cost is a factor. I interviewed three doulas and I chose the one that cost the least because I was on a budget having been laid off. I also didn't see a reason why I should pay over $1000 for less than eight hours of work. Some of the doulas just had a flat cost for birth that was in the $2000-$3000 range, and didn't have a special package for planned C-section. That just didn't make a whole lot of sense to me because planned C-section is a world apart from vaginal birth or vaginal birth converted to emergency C-section. Both of those experiences take much longer than a planned C-section.

I did two interviews with the doula I ended up choosing, and though she was very positive, what I found out later was that she is autistic. As a high-functioning autistic person, she sometimes was not able to really read the room and consistently react in a soothing way. This seems obvious, but only if you know the person is autistic beforehand. She spoke so authoritatively in our interviews that I didn't catch it. After the baby was born, and we were transported to our little hospital room where we could receive visitors, there were a few little awkward moments because she might be speaking too loudly for the room or getting herself worked up about a hypothetical topic that had not yet happened. It really was mostly about her tone, and mild inability to consistently react in an emotionally empathetic way even though she understood what was happening from an emotional standpoint. It was odd. I could see that my family was puzzled and even a bit put off, but even those moments did not override the fact that I was grateful to have put someone in place to do what I needed. It was really eating at me to know that I was going to be cut open and incapacitated at the point of my child's birth and not even be able to interact with him for sometime after he was born. To her credit, she showed up completely on time, in her doula uniform with her doula credentials totally ready to do her job. I just should have looked at more than three people.

Some of the questions I asked the doulas were, had they worked at my hospital before? I was curious to know if they had any relationships there with the doctors and nurses already. I wanted to know how many C-sections they had been a part of. Had they ever had a C-section themselves? I wanted to make sure they were super clear on the birth plan for the baby and all of the medicines that are generally administered to the baby after birth. But again, I was so focused on cost that I let some nagging in my gut go by unaddressed. Don't make my mistake. The mood of the room is everything during childbirth.

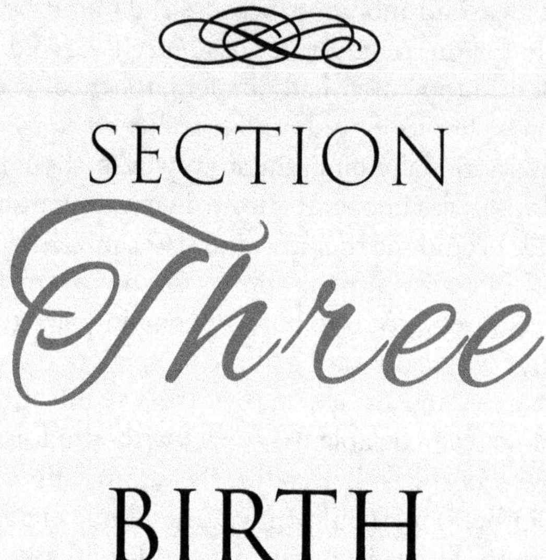

SECTION Three

BIRTH

What I Brought With Me

The hospital where I delivered is extremely busy for maternity. They deliver more babies annually than any other community hospital in the United States, so I did my best to make sure that everything was taken care of ahead of time so that we had a smooth experience. After my doctor said that she had scheduled the surgery, I made a note for myself to call the hospital about a week before the scheduled date to ensure that I was on the operating room schedule for that day. I made sure that they had my insurance information. Then, I started planning. What I was going to bring? I was very nervous about coming home alone with the baby after having had this surgery. I was planning to stay in the hospital for as long as possible after birth. I packed a couple of pajama sets with the shirt that buttons down so that I could easily breastfeed and do skin to skin. I never used them at the hospital though. I wore the hospital gowns the entire time. I had read all about staying hydrated and eating enough so that you can produce milk. So I brought my nut bar snacks from Costco. I brought a cooler that had my Body Armor drinks because I had read that women had good success producing milk from drinking them. I brought approximately 6 outfits for the baby. I brought my computer of course, which is like an appendage that I can't live without. I brought my own Tylenol and Advil, the big humongo size bottles that I had again, purchased at Costco. I of course brought my Doona car seat/stroller combo. I brought my camera tripod and my Canon which I also never used. I did all the photo and video capturing from my phone. It felt like I had brought enough to move in, and I cannot stress enough, most of that stuff I did not use. I was so busy learning how to take care of my son that I didn't have time or the inclination to do multiple outfit changes for myself, and all that sort of nonsense.

The Main Event

I had read a lot of pregnancy message boards and heard all about getting the epidural and how painful it was. I think it helped that I could not see what was going on. The fact that they're behind your back doing whatever it is they're doing, and also the fact that I had prepared my mind for any level of pain, made it not so bad when he inserted the needle in my back. It was uncomfortable for sure, but it was bearable. I remember my anesthesiologist and my doula being really surprised at how I reacted. After that, things began to move very quickly. I laid there on my side for what seemed like ten minutes and then, they flipped me to my back and we started wheeling into the operating room. By this time I was well and truly nervous and starting to feel nauseous, frankly. I was most nervous that I was going to throw up and choke while I was on my back, or that I would be heaving so much as to interrupt the abdomen cutting. Both were extremely terrible options in my mind so I kept asking if I could be tilted to sit up some more and they said flatly, no. Now that I think about it, it makes sense. They could hardly give me a good incision if I am sitting up, but at the moment, I was in a panic, so obviously not thinking straight. My doctor came in immediately after that, we said our "hey girl heys", and she got to work. She was pulling my son out within minutes. Being cut open was not terrible, it just felt like pressure, and then, voila! There was a little boy! The sewing shut however, I will say was breathtakingly painful. I know that there had been some adjusting on the epidural medicine when I was complaining about feeling nauseous. So maybe I didn't have enough medicine in me to not feel the sewing, but I certainly felt *every* stitch. They brought the baby over and showed him to me while this was going on. I can only imagine they do this as a distraction from the pain, but I could barely greet my little guy. I remember looking at him and thinking, "wow he's so cute, he has lips like mine!" and also thinking, "God that really hurts!" I thought I was going to faint. That's how painful it was.

First Night With No Support Person and Pain Management

One thing I didn't consider was the first night in the hospital and the fact that, even though there is medical staff coming in every hour, I still would be by myself. I am not sure what I was thinking. I hired the doula and I knew that the doula wasn't spending the night. But I just hadn't really thought too deeply about needing anyone to be there with me overnight. Frankly, I was eager to be alone with my child, and talk to him. I wasn't thinking about having someone to hand him to me, or helping me reach the diapers which were under his bassinet in the middle of the night while newly recuperating from surgery. The nurses aren't really around when you need someone to help you grab the baby out of the bassinet, and some of them will be put off if you ask them to do tasks that are outside of their purview. A friend had asked me if I wanted her to come and stay with me in the hospital, and I told her no. That was a mistake. It is good to have someone, especially that first night to stay with you in the hospital because you're freaking out about being someone's mom, feeling shock, anxiety and pain and literally just trying to hold it together.

I remember being upset when nurses would come in to check his vitals, and then place the bassinet at weird angles, far away from my bed when they could clearly see that I was in the room alone and had had a C-section that day. Trying to scoot myself to the side of the bed where the bassinet is, then having to reach up to pick him up, you're having to use a lot of your abdominal muscles for these activities. I also had a nurse also make me feel bad about it when I checked in. She said incredulously to me, "you don't have anyone staying here with you overnight!?" and I felt shamed. Surely I'm not the first single mother or the last, at this hospital. As I already stated, this is the busiest community hospital in the whole United States. And yes, I did make a mistake not having someone there with me, but I managed so obviously it is doable.

The main thing that saved me that first night was that I was still on epidural medicine, so I didn't feel the pain as acutely. But within the first 24 hours, they cut those meds off. They said I could have Tylenol and Ibuprofen, and told me to ask for morphine pills when I felt the pain ratcheting upward. Now, if you wait until you feel pain to ask for a painkiller that comes in pill form, by the time it kicks in, you feel like you want to die. And that was what was happening to me. There was not a good plan in place for my pain management. I was surprised because even though I know many times black women are treated as though we have an unusually high threshold for pain, I still had just experienced a C-section that day! I could not fathom why anyone thought a few Tylenol, Ibuprofen and a random morphine pill here and there would be sufficient! By the middle of that second day, I was ready to cuss a few folks out. Knowing that I planned to stay at least 4 days at the hospital I struggled to put on a smile and pull myself together enough to let the nurses know that if we did not get this pain management together in quick order it was not going to be good. We ended up discontinuing the morphine completely. I was prescribed Percocet which was the same painkiller I was given the year previous after my myomectomy. When I took them before, they managed my pain wonderfully for the first 4 days and then I didn't need them anymore. I asked for the same protocol that I had then, and once we got that in place everything was fine. I knew that I needed to stay ahead of the pain because it was vitally important that I be as present as possible to take care of my son. I committed to myself and I committed to him.

So after I got my pain management schedule locked in, I stuck to it religiously.

Exposed

I was also not prepared for how helpless and exposed I felt when the nurse came in to take out the epidural about 12 hours after surgery. I think I stared at her blankly for a few seconds when she told me to walk to the bathroom and use it in front of her. I don't think I've peed in front of anyone in 25 years. Back then, on a drunken party night where you and a girlfriend go to the restroom together to gossip, we might plop down on the throne and pee in front of each other. Certainly not since then, so that was very embarrassing for me, but of course, the nurses see this every day. This particular nurse was super encouraging and she also was extremely kind. She was the nicest of all of the nurses that I had, so if I had to pee in front of anyone, thank God, it was her.

Even knowing ahead of time that I planned to breastfeed, the amount of times I was having to whip out my breast in front of family members, to try to get the breast feeding going, also threw me for a loop. You don't have quite enough time to be embarrassed, but it's still there. Underneath the overwhelm is just a complete sense of exposure, so who you choose to have around you in those moments is of critical importance.

Breastfeeding

Breastfeeding was a surprise. After I got sewn up and went into recovery, they brought the baby over to me immediately to allow him to breastfeed. He tried suckling for about 20 minutes but then began to cry because nothing was coming out. They took him off of me and put him in his own little bassinet, and we stayed in recovery for about an hour or so before we went into our room. But it became clear throughout the day that although he was suckling, he wasn't getting any milk, and he was crying because he was hungry. He was also having a problem latching because he had a lip tie. I was confused about what to do. I had a lot of information coming at me about it from many different people. When I looked into it, it looked like it meant a laser surgery for him, which I didn't want to do. He seemed to feed from a bottle just fine so I didn't see why we needed to do anything else. There was one moment where the limits of my grace gave out at the end of the first day where one of the nurses came in and was noticing that his latch was not perfect. The nurse kept forcing him onto the nipple, and she was very forceful in pushing his little soft head. She did it two or three times and after that third time I snapped at her. It was just a reflexive instinct. I didn't like the way she was grabbing his head, considering he was only about 10 hours old. There are lots of reasons why the breastfeeding process may not be happening perfectly on day one. There is no need to stress mom and baby out throwing every theory and "solution" in mom's face, or forcing baby onto the nipple. We ended up feeding him a pre-made Similac preemie formula there in the hospital which I also was not overjoyed about but, I didn't have a choice because my milk wasn't coming in yet. As we all know, fed is best.

Somehow, I didn't understand going into this experience that I was going to have to pump every 2 hours, even though I was not seeing any milk, then get out of bed, wash and dry all the little pump parts in addition to feeding him every 2 hours from the pre-made bottle. I knew that you don't get any sleep once the baby arrives, and I was prepared for that, but I wasn't prepared for hopping in and out of the bed while dealing with the incision and all of the pumping and related activities. It took at least a week and the Mother's Milk tea from Traditional Medicinals for my milk to actually come in. And when it did, it still didn't come in like gangbusters. So I was mixing a few ounces of breastmilk into the formula for the first few months to help boost his immunity. But frankly, the whole pumping every 2 hours, I was not able to manage. If I did 4 to 6 sessions in a day, I was doing well, but then I would fall down on feeding and hydrating myself which was working against the pumping. Between trying to work and take care of him, I did not have the wherewithal for the constant pumping sessions. That was one thing that I had not wrapped my brain around regarding what that meant for life and time and schedules.

Lack of Sleep

As I said, I was prepared for lack of sleep. Having recently been in the hospital for the myomectomy, I knew that the nurses tend to come in every hour to take vitals, talk to you and give you medicines so I was prepared for that. I had set my alarms for every two hours as well for diapers changes and feeding. I was just so obsessed with the baby that I wanted to stay up and watch him. I could not relax enough to sleep. I was running on adrenaline and that adrenaline carried me through probably the first two months of his life. I just did not sleep. My anxiety was through the roof which we'll talk about later in this book. But between my adrenaline and my anxiety, sleep was pretty much the last thing on my agenda.

Length of Hospital Stay

Normally the hospital tries to throw you out quickly as we all know, and as patients, we also try to rush out because no one wants to stay in the hospital longer than they have to and the cost of it can be completely prohibitive. But in this case, I had plans to stay at least 3 or 4 days. I wanted to stay as long as I possibly could so that I could learn how to take care of the baby with some oversight. One of my doctors came in, and he agreed with me that I should stay if it would make me more comfortable. So I did just what he suggested. I stayed from Wednesday morning to Sunday afternoon. At that point, the baby who had arrived a few weeks early was stabilized. I could move around sufficiently, and the baby and I were beginning to get into our own little rhythm.

SECTION *Four*

FOURTH TRIMESTER THOSE FIRST MONTHS POSTPARTUM

Postpartum Anxiety/Hormones

Secondary to the fact that black women suffer the most maternal death in hospitals, I was also concerned about postpartum depression especially after having experienced that little bout of depression before coming off of the IVF hormones in the first trimester. I was aware that my hormones were certainly going to be fluctuating up and down after the baby was born. The whole process of actually giving birth, the speed of it, the amount of information coming at me, and the new responsibilities created a very overwhelming experience.

My anxiety set in on the second day. The first day I was just excited and happy to hold him and praise the Lord, but the second day I was like, "OK. How do I take care of this baby?" My anxiety levels went through the roof. I had real fears about earning enough to take care of him which was rather ridiculous because I had resources and I work in sales which means I can always get a job. But yet I still had what could be viewed as an unreasonable fear about providing. I also had an unreasonable fear about someone taking him out of my room even though he had a bracelet on his ankle that matched my hospital bracelet. When the nurses would come to take him to his pediatrician appointments in the nursery, I was reluctant to let them take him without me. I literally shuffled down the hall, rolling my IV pole on day two to follow him to his appointment and stare at him through the nursery window. You should have seen the looks I was getting from the nurses. But my mind was overwhelmed with what "might" happen. My hormone fluctuation was also contributing to me having violent shivering attacks. The temperature in my hospital room was very comfortable but I was literally teeth chattering and shivering like I was at the North Pole. I was piling on the blankets and covers as high as a mountain. When I looked up that symptom, I found that it was due to an effect of fluid or heat loss and hormonal changes in the body after giving birth.

I told my OB about how I was feeling, which is where anyone feeling this way should start, but I also started looking online for what kind of supplements I could take to manage my moods and hormones postpartum. I found a postpartum pill on Amazon that had regular vitamins in it, but it also had ashwagandha in it for mood support. I began taking it and I started feeling better almost immediately. I still had thoughts about earning and being able to handle everything, but it was nowhere near the almost crippling fear that I had before. Those first two weeks I cried a few minutes every day just because of the overload of emotions: happiness, fear, overwhelm. I'm not a huge crier but I am an *extremely* emotional person so with my hormones out of whack, it's no wonder that I was experiencing these intense emotions. The pills for me, really did help but we should bear in mind that other women may need some prescription help from their doctors. What worked for me is not going to work for everyone. Also, the full solve for me was two fold. The second part was, I had to start watching and listening to things that were going to make me feel better. I began watching travel bloggers on YouTube that would post these fabulous videos of far-flung places like the Maldives set to very soothing music. With my 55 inch tv displaying glossy views of the Indian Ocean, I felt like I too was in the Maldives, which was an amazing feeling. Also, getting back into my personal development and mindset work helped to remind me that my current circumstances, even as fantastic as they were, were not the end of my story and that I still had so much more to build and create. Actively taking back control of my thoughts really helped me to climb out of the anxiety that was trying to grab ahold of me.

Visitors

I honestly wasn't sure if I was going to have many visitors, but my son was born during the holiday season. So of the folks that did come, there certainly were those who had been running through Hartsfield International Airport, the busiest airport on the planet, and then wanting to come by to see my baby. People carry germs. That's just life. I try not to get too freaked out about it, but with my son, I definitely wanted to protect him as much as I could until he was able to start his immunity protocols which is not until about 2 months of life. So, my plan for visitors was to have them wear masks. I am not a fan of masking in general, but for newborns I am. I didn't want people breathing on my baby. Period. I also asked for them to wash their hands and use hand sanitizer afterward. Then, they could interact with the baby. There also was a rule of no kissing, which should go without saying. Of course, we had some push back within our little community, but I stuck to my guns. My baby, my rules, no debate.

Finding A Pediatrician

I began looking for a pediatrician for the baby when I first got to our new location. I had already identified a doctor for him when I thought I was staying in New Jersey who had a sort of membership set-up where you could get in to see him or get a phone call from him pretty much at any time if you were a part of his membership. I liked that type of concierge service. But with us moving I had to start over. I started looking into the pediatricians near my area and quickly I was happy to find one. He didn't have the membership type service but he is very flexible with his patients and parents and has been in the community for 25 years. He answered all of my questions about allergies, immunology and formulas. He was attentive to our needs and did not dismiss us at all. I have heard some horror stories about pediatricians that can be quite authoritarian and dismissive towards parental concerns, even going as far as to throw families out of the practice, and that's definitely not the type of practice that I wanted to be involved with.

Getting My Body Back

Spoiler alert, it's not back. I've never had body or health issues other than the reproductive issues I've outlined in this book. I've never had any problems with body image except for when I was a teenager and I started getting hips. I didn't understand that it was a good thing until much later. But that's a story for another day! After leaving the hospital, my entire body was was incredibly swollen, especially my legs and feet. I was very concerned. I'd never seen my feet look like this. My feet have always been skinny and bony; but then, my lower extremities looked like an elephant's. I could barely move them but everyone kept saying that it was normal from all of the fluids that had been pumped into me at the hospital. I still hated to see it though. It really messed with my head. It took a few weeks for the swelling to go down.

As for overall recovery, I had mistakenly equated the recovery from the myomectomy surgery of the previous year with recovery from a C-section. They are in no way the same thing. I was not really prepared for the incision discomfort that goes on for months. Even now, I am six months out from the C-section and I still have discomfort in the incision area from time to time if the baby kicks me in the stomach or inadvertently steps on it. The scar tissue is not yet completely healed. I have always had very strong abdominal muscles and now my stomach is flabby, but it's nothing that 2 to 3 good months of being on a Pilates reformer can't fix. Of course, one would have to find the time to get on that reformer and also have the money to do so. Finding the time and discipline to get back to my old body has been challenging because I am seated much of the day in the house.

I find that when I approach this plan of getting my body back from a perspective of youthful longevity and being here for my son for the next 50 years, there's more impetus and urgency to do it. I was doing way more movement when I was first cleared for exercise at two months postpartum by my doctor than I have been lately. I started doing a pilates mat in the bedroom while the baby was sleeping and I hadn't really gone back to working full force. I find that now post pregnancy, my body is less forgiving. It tells on me with everything I eat and every exercise I don't do. I once had the opportunity to meet basketball legend Michael Jordan's personal trainer, Tim Grover, decades ago when I was still in college. I was moaning about the fact that I couldn't have pizza, because I was aspiring to be a model and stay at a certain weight. I'll never forget what he said to me. He said, "it's less about what you don't do and more about what you do do", and I never forgot that. Meaning, it's the workouts and the movement, and the weight training that are gonna bring the results, not denying myself a slice of pizza. And when you think about it, it's true.

When I do workout, I focus on my core muscles. Not just because I want flat abs or I want to get rid of the mommy shelf where the incision is, but because it's helpful to have a strong core when you're lifting heavy car seats and strollers. Even just carrying the baby around in my arms can be challenging when I'm not regularly working out and pushing my body to the limit.

Drifting away from food and diet disciplines once you have a baby is easy to do. I have people that bring me cakes and cookies and all sorts of treats saying that I deserve it. And of course, I do but within moderation. I've always been a coffee fanatic, but I developed an even stronger dependence and addiction to coffee after my son was born. However, it is incredibly dehydrating and it was working against my milk production. I was telling myself that I deserved it because I had to get up every two hours. I needed it to get my work done. I didn't really need excuses, but I could have come up with a book of excuses for why I should be drinking more than one cup of coffee per day. So that's an addiction that even now I'm still battling unsuccessfully, but happily. I also found that I was drinking a lot more sugar soda which I never used to do before I got pregnant. I developed a habit of drinking Fanta while pregnant. That's a habit that I haven't completely put down yet either. It's curious how little things can sneak their way in and seem harmless at first, but can become insidious and cause massive inflammation if not put in check. So I know I have to keep an eye on these new habits and cravings that did not used to exist before the baby.

Post Pregnancy Supplements

I took the postpartum mood pill for about 3 months. I'm also still taking my prenatal pill. It's packed with so many vitamins and minerals that the body needs that I don't see any reason to stop taking it. I began to add back in my pre-pregnancy youthful longevity supplements like the omega 3, chlorophyll, and CoQ10. I also took this opportunity to address the estrogen and progesterone deficiencies in my body due to menopause. So now I take phytoestrogen supplements. I also use progesterone cream two weeks out of the month, so I'll do two weeks of phytoestrogens alone. Then I do two weeks of phytoestrogens plus progesterone cream and I've been feeling pretty normal, with thankfully no mood issues.

Accepting Help

I've been the queen of, "I'll do it myself", pretty much my entire life. Do for self, was a big phrase in my household growing up. So I've never been a person who was good at asking for help. When you first have a baby, of course, everyone wants to help you. Now, I'm no fool. I know that it is more about the baby than me, but I was smart enough to get over feeling like a burden to others and just force myself to say yes to people offering to bring food by, or offering to watch the baby for a few hours while I go grocery shopping because I knew I needed help! I had committed to taking this baby journey alone so I had no expectations of help. When you have no expectations of help and help starts coming in, the inclination is always going to be to say no. Fight that inclination with all of your might, and say yes. Receive the help. You can move faster that way. Take advantage, while the baby is cute and a magnet for everyone. Now is the time to enlist their aid and lock them in as a part of his village!

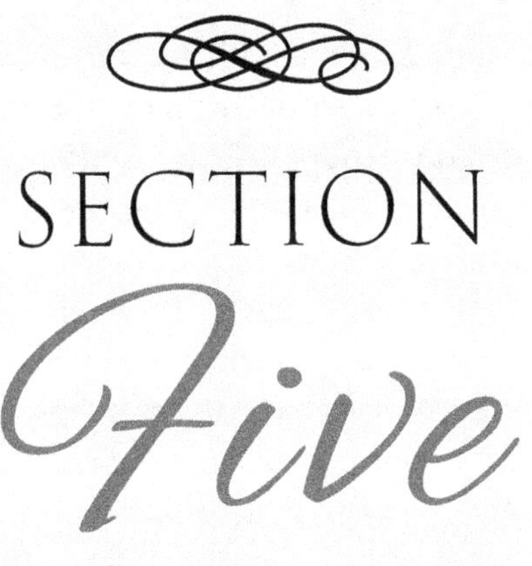

SECTION
Five

SETTLING INTO THE NEW NORMAL

What Is "The New Normal"?

Since my child is only 6 months at the time of this writing, we still do not have a "normal" yet. Some things that we do are scheduled like bath time and meals. But he still doesn't have a very strict schedule for his sleep. I decided I was not going to go back and forth with him on that at this point in time because he couldn't even understand what it was that I was trying to say to him. I guess my "new normal" is throwing out the window the somewhat rigid ways that I used to live by before. Work, personal development and family time all morph together. I knew going in that I was going to have to be more efficient. I was prepared to be better at delegating and trusting other people to do tasks because I just can't do everything myself anymore, nor do I even want to. I still have to psych myself up to hand off a task though. It's such a compulsive thing, a constant repentance to ruthlessly go through my activities and start getting rid of those that are taking time away from the most important activities, which are to parent and produce revenue.

Before I had a child, I always strived to live a great life and have great experiences. Now, I want to have great experiences and share that with my child. It's fun being able to introduce him to things like his music class, going to the zoo, reading books and visiting different places around our city. Of course, he has no idea what any of this is now, but he will and it's just my hope that he'll say, "I had a great childhood thanks to my mom". It's such a change to have my own family now. It was incredible on Christmas to wake up and not be by myself in the house. I watched the Super Bowl with a 2 month old. I watch Formula 1 on race weekends with a baby. My baby. I love that this is my "new normal".

Back To Work With or Without Full Time Care

I only took about two complete weeks off of work after my son was born. So my new normal in terms of work has been very long workdays. During the week, I don't separate family time from work time because he's always with me. I take fun breaks from working on marketing to read him a book or play with him on his playmat. Eventually, I plan to have someone come in and be a nanny to him while I work from home but we are not there yet. I've been fortunate that I've not had to rush back into a very rigid work situation. I realize that not everyone has that luxury. And I'm also really fortunate that I have family members nearby who are eager to watch him when I need help. These past six months, I considered to be maternity leave even though I'm working for myself. This is why I definitely see the value in women deploying whatever sort of business they can manage for themselves. Generating new income streams is important to the freedom we seek in raising our children in the ways we think are best.

Keeping Up With Friends

Like most new moms, I've not been great about keeping up with every detail of my friends' lives. But I do try to reach out, sending photos and updates. I have grown to hate social media, but it is a necessary evil. I jump on a few times a week to post on business accounts and sometimes will take that opportunity to show love to friends on my personal one. However, the random meetings at the bar, and fancy dinners for the heck of it every week are long gone. I'm not sad about it either. It's a savings on my wallet, but I definitely want to maintain my friendships. I've had some of these friends for 30 years. The ways of connecting are just different now. I hope that sending long texts to let them know I'm thinking about them allows people understand that they are still important to me and that even though I am now "Mom", I'm also still Kia. I didn't trade one persona for the other. I'm not trying to morph into super-mom with a giant Stanley cup going to Mommy and Me groups all day long. I see my new life as augmenting my old one. I hope that my friends see it that way too. But if they don't, I know they will let me know!

Mom Guilt

It's amazing how much mom guilt you can feel especially when you're working next to your child, which I do a lot. I dictate emails with him on my lap. He's sitting next to me as I'm working on this book, and I sometimes feel guilty, giving him toys and then typing for 20 minutes. However, he's not going to remember this time when he is older. And also, I am working with him on educational things. Literally everything is educational when you are six months old. God has blessed us with a great life, and even in that, I still sometimes feel guilty.

People tried to make me feel guilty that I hadn't started him on rice cereal at a certain point in time, even down to the lady police officer we met on the street one day. Then when I started him on cereal, I chose organic oatmeal instead of rice, and people tried to make me feel guilty about that. Then people tried to make me feel guilty about not giving him certain table foods yet. "When was he gonna be eating this food? And when is he gonna eat that food?", like you don't have enough things going on in your mind between working and bills to be worried about how many fruits and vegetables a six-month-old has sampled. I usually just say we're working on it and give a tight lipped smile. And hopefully from my demeanor, people know to "back back". Respectfully.

It's not productive to entertain guilty thoughts. It's never great to focus on what's lacking, especially when there's so much here that is good. A healthy, happy child is priceless in any context, but especially this one. I believe that guilty thoughts are not our own. They are thoughts that come to torture, thoughts that come to annoy us, thoughts that come to harass, and we have to cast those thoughts down and make a decision to think right thoughts and have a right mind. That's really where my own personal development work comes in. I know that I have to constantly be feeding myself the right information in order to keep my life and by extension, my son's life progressing and moving forward.

Final Learnings

God told Adam and Eve to be fruitful and multiply (Genesis 1:28), but He didn't put many qualifiers on it. There was nothing mentioned about age. At the moment, I don't have an Adam. Adam might be coming later, who knows? But I'm glad that God chose me to be able to participate in the multiplication and I intend to honor it every day. When things look bleak and you have no idea how a problem can be solved, God knows how the problem can be solved. He always has a ram in the bush. He is a powerful problem solver, if only we will wholeheartedly engage in the exercise of stepping out on faith. My journey has been one faith step after another. Going from faith to faith feels a little bit like surfing. You're flying and constantly trying to find your balance. You're constantly taking in new information, processing it and reacting to it. This has been one of the deepest learning curves I've ever encountered, but it's been the one with the biggest payoff. I'm fortunate, blessed and happy every day. And that's really the reason why I wrote this book. For as much as I know about health and wellness and the body, I didn't know that I could do this in the way that I did it. I wanted to share that information with others and hopefully inspire other women to go for the same happiness that I am currently experiencing. I send my best to you, Dear Reader, no matter what choices you make or how your journey winds and turns. I hope that the one thing you walk away with from this book is the value in going from faith to faith and believing that your desired end is already yours.

RESOURCES

IVF Clinics

*Find real reviews of any IVF doctor and clinic: Fertility IQ, https://www.fertilityiq.com/

*Sama – IVF "Care From Anywhere", https://www.sama.life/

Embryo Adoption

*Embryo Adoption Awareness Center List Of Clinics With Embryo Donation Programs By State: https://embryoadoption.org/clinic-donation-programs/

*Facebook Embryo Adoption and Donation Support Group: https://www.facebook.com/groups/EmbryoAdoption/

*Facebook Christian Embryo Adoption: https://www.facebook.com/groups/1847954242090254/

*California Conceptions Donor Embryo Program (CA and beyond): https://californiaconceptions.com/

*Atlantic Shared Beginnings Donor Eggs and Embryos (NC and beyond): https://sharedbeginnings.life/embryo-programs-atlantic-shared-beginnings/

*Embryo Donation International (FL, don't have many African-American embryos): https://www.embryodonation.com/home.php

*Embryo Solution (WI): https://www.embryosolution.com/embryo-adoption

Pre Pregnancy Supplement List

Omega 3 liquid form

CoQ10 liquid form

Chlorophyll

Magnesium powder

Vitamin B

Vitamin D

Zinc

Westab prenatal (doctor prescribed)

Iron liquid form (because my red blood count was low)

Cats Claw (because my white blood count was low)

Copper
*Action-Fertility Acupuncture

Questions To Ask The Potential Doctors On Your Team

Questions For A Myomectomy Surgeon

1. Is this your primary activity: fibroid surgeries, endometriosis surgeries?

2. How long have you been performing them?

3. How many surgeries have you performed for my specific condition, intramuscular, exterior, interior, x number of fibroids, etc.

4. How will you perform the surgery, what kind of incision, robotic or not?

5. How long is my recovery?

6. Will I be able to carry a baby afterwards?

7. Do you have testimonials from previous patients?

8. What was your most complicated case?

Questions For An IVF Doctor

1. Do they work with single women (if you are single)?

2. Do they work with women who are my age?

3. Is there a cut off age that they won't work with?

4. What would the possible complications be for me?

5. Do you see any fibroids that have come back or any obstructions to implantation?

6. Any questions around readings from your CBC bloodwork that do not fall in the normal ranges

Questions For An OB-GYN or MFM

1. Have they delivered a baby for someone your age?

2. What sort of problems or conditions will they be keeping an eye out for?

3. What is their delivery plan?

4. Will they definitely be the person to deliver?

5. Will the OB and MFM both be present for delivery?

Questions For A Doula

1. Have they worked at the hospital where you will deliver? Do they have any relationships with the doctors and nurses there?

2. How many C-sections, emergency C-sections, VBACS etc. have they been a part of?

3. How many children do they have? Had they ever had a C-section themselves?

4. Do they have any issues with your birth plan?

5. How do they deal with stressful situations?

Questions For A Pediatrician

1. How soon can we test for allergies?

2. What formulas do you recommend? What do you think about the formula I would like to use?

3. Are you flexible on shot schedules?

4. What experience do you have and resources do you use for autistic children?

Things To Consider When Hiring Childcare

1. Create your ad and narrow down your list to 5 to 10 people to interview at a coffee shop or park so they don't have to visit your home before the background check.

2. Be very clear about what the rate of pay will be in your ad, and don't negotiate.

3. Be very clear about your expectations for what you want them to do in terms of housework, laundry and play/ teaching with the child.

Influencer Journeys

Simply Tanika: Female Fertility https://www.simplytanika.com/

FOOLING MY FERTILITY & EXPECTING AT 50

Influencer Journeys

Simply Tanika: Female Fertility https://www.simplytanika.com/

ACKNOWLEDGEMENTS

All praise to The Most High God and to Yeshua my Lord and Savior. I can't do anything without His Grace, and I take no glory in the events of my life, all glory goes to God.

Thank you to my wonderful physicians who have been a part of my team at some point in the journey, Dr. I. Stacey Anand, Dr. Allen Morgan, Dr. Robin Hilsenrath, Dr. Raymond Allen, Dr. Meir Olcha, Dr. Ulas Bozdogan, Dr. Michael Dresdner.

Thank you to my family who packed, cooked, kept watch and generally supported: Sabree, Aunt LaVerne, Malir, Conisha, Robert, Darryl, Margo, Amyr and Jennifer, Malik, Abu, Sheana, Aunt Shirley, Uncle Greg and Ms. Theda. Thank you to my girls who supported and kept me sane: Edith, Zeki, Nancy, Star, Natalie, Kim S.S., Megan B., Kemba, Honor, Adolpha, Rachael and Alisha but a special thank you to Dr. Kai Pittman who held my hand every day on my journey to impart all of her recent wisdom. Thank you to my Hearts who showed up and have been supporting since 1991, LA, Samine, Brigette, Kym S., Katina, Rhonda, Dilsey, Paula, and Tosca. To my play brothers Josh, Adam and Justin M. who are always on time with levity and a male perspective. I love all y'all!

Thank you to the Mature Mama and Single Mother By Choice influencers who transparently shared their stories via social media and kept me inspired, specifically, Simply Tanika whose thoroughness in sharing her journey is unmatched.

ABOUT THE AUTHOR

Kia Glover is a music tech founder, sales leader, songwriter and performer who finally broke free of the mental paradigm that welcoming a baby into her family had to look or happen a certain way. In addition to her music-centered projects, she is focused on living a life of celebrated Youthful Longevity and building a community around the best methods and products for living long and strong (on Instagram and YouTube @myyouthfullongevity).

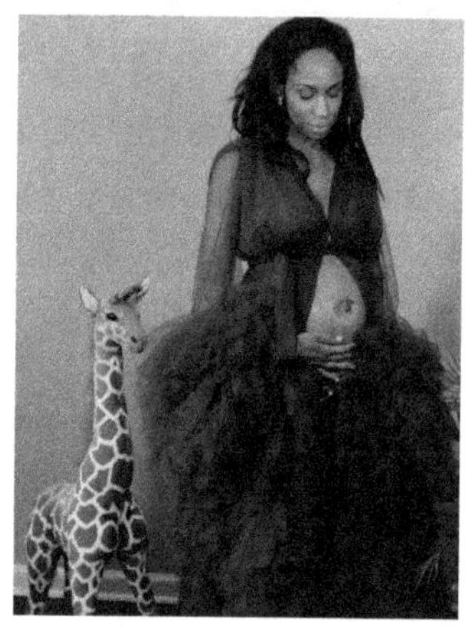

9 798990 993020